HOME-MADE SANITIZER

How to make quality Sanitizer at Home

Save Money by Making Quality Sanitizers at Home and kill all Viruses and Bacteria

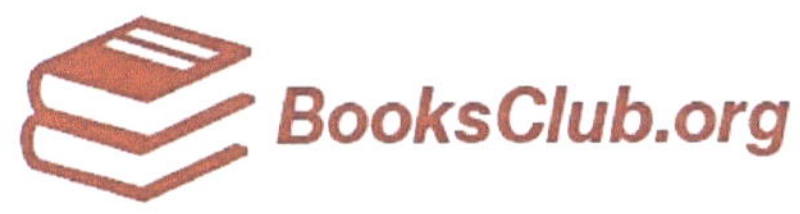

Table of Content

INTRODUCTION

Owing to the fast spread of the novel coronavirus (nCoV), which gives birth to the coronavirus disease 2019 (COVID-19), the market for hand sanitizers has been significant as the item can be used to destroy up to 99 percent of the virus on human bodies and other surfaces. Sellers, both locally and online, have abused the product's high demand to raise its price to unprecedented levels. Therefore, learning how to manufacture a high-quality hand sanitizer at home and cut out unnecessary expenses has become essential. Hand sanitizers may be used to destroy most pathogens, including coronavirus, on the hand before touching the nose, eyes, or mouth with the same finger and being infected with the virus.

Besides the coronavirus issue, it's strongly recommended that you sanitize your hands whenever you touch objects that may have been infected with germs. A hand sanitizer comes straight to the aid every time. The item can be carried away in a small bottle or container. The Center for Disease Control (CDC) and the World Health Organization (WHO) recommend that a hand sanitizer must include at least 60 percent alcohol, which is adequate to destroy germs and persistent viruses such as the novel coronavirus on any surface within 60 seconds; the primary component of the mixture is alcohol.

Towards this end, this book includes hand sanitizer recipes to manufacture a sanitizer at home or full scale. You will be educated about everything that you need to know about creating a high-quality home-made hand sanitizer, plus viruses that the hand sanitizer cannot destroy.

The book also guides how to make Aloe-Vera gel, which is also a primary ingredient required to make a hand sanitizer. So start reading and educate yourself to stay protected.

Chapter 1: Understanding the Basics

1.1 What is Sanitizer?

Sanitizers are typically used to eliminate bacteria and viruses on the surface of the hands or body. They are generally available as consistency in a gel, but they are also available in the form of lotions, liquid sprays, and foams. Necessary contact time with antimicrobial agents while using hand sanitizer is required. Many sanitizers comprise around 65 percent to 85 percent isopropyl or ethyl alcohol combined with water and gels such as glycol and glycerin to avoid drying out the skin of the con-

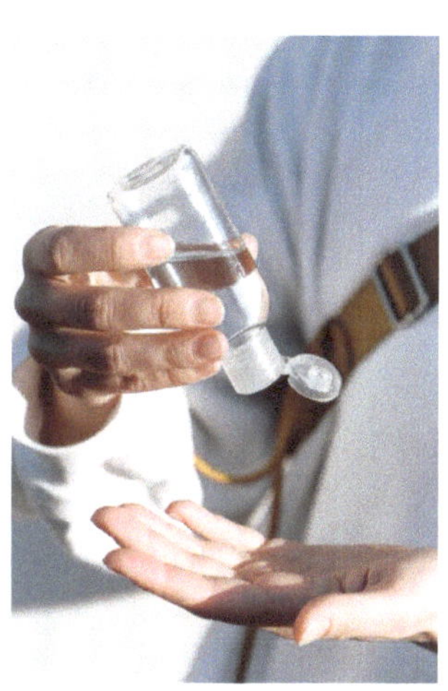

sumers. The item resulting is usually sold in a hand gel or liquid spray under brand name products. Hand sanitizers reliant on alcohol are superior in most health-care environments over handwashing with soap and water. Possible explanations include it is easy to use anytime and quite portable. However, handwashing with soap and water should be practiced if contamination can be observed, e.g., after use of the toilet, it should be performed. Currently, in the outbreak of the SARS-COV-2 Virus, alcohol-based hand sanitizers are in demand, and to meet decontamination criteria, water-based hand sanitizers containing chlorine are sufficient.

1.2 Need for a Sanitizer in today's World

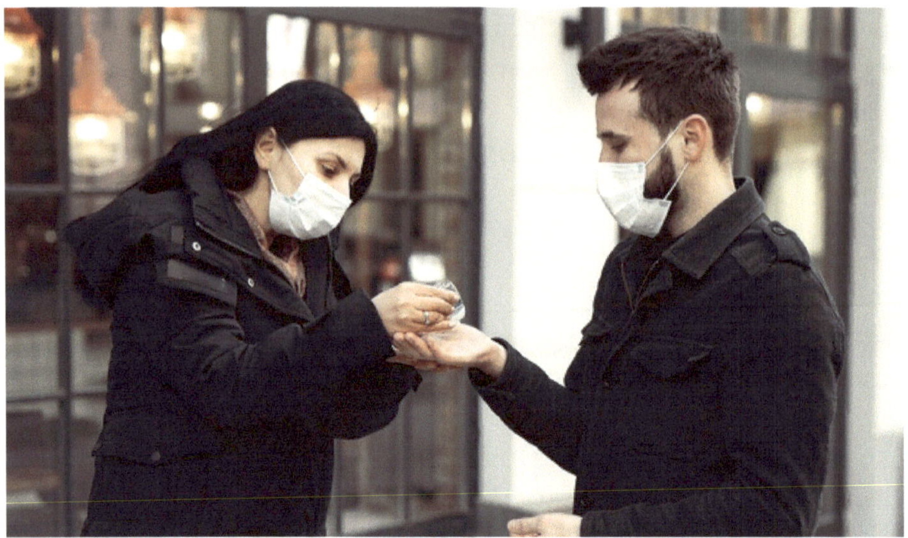

Sanitizers are a necessity for this century, as each year comes with a new collection of viral epidemics, they are essential to avoid spreading them. Basic hygiene is of paramount importance in these situations, and hand sanitizers are a recommended way of keeping the hands safe from germs. An individual cannot wash his hands all the time; however, he can easily use those gel-like liquids. Kids, in particular, should be forced to use the sanitizers to maintain their hands clean before eating something. Bacteria and viruses can make you sick from the hands and objects we handle during our daily activities. Hand disinfectants based alcohol do not kill all forms of bacteria, including gastric worms called norovirus, certain parasites, and clostridium difficile, which cause extreme diarrhea. However, hand sanitizing can surely reduce the number of bacteria, viruses, and fungicides on your hands.

In hospital emergency rooms, pre and post visiting friends and family, you should wash your hands. If detergent and water are not accessible, use a hand sanitizer based alcohol, which contains at least 65 percent alcohol and wash it with water and soap as soon as it is available. Surveys show that one in five people do not regularly wash their hands—68 percent of those who do not use detergent. Providing hand disinfectants in sensitive areas increases the probability of people destroying dangerous bacteria. The American Journal of Infection Control (AJIC) study showed that encouraging the use of hand disinfectants in schools decreased absenteeism by approximately 25%.

1.3 Comparing Hand Sanitizer with other Disinfectants

After the pandemic, everyone has some form of disinfectant in their pocket, on their desk, and in their car. But how effective are such hand sanitizers, especially wipes? Will our hand sanitizer cloths work? Although manufacturers of disinfectants say that most wipes kill 99.9 percent of harmful viruses and bacteria, this has not always been the case. These are mostly tested on inanimate objects, not on human bodies, so they don't kill a lot of dangerous viruses. The easiest way for everyone to stay safe is to wash their hands with soap and water. If they are not available, hand sanitizers are best than not washing your hands. Some claim that increased use of cloths and gels to clean hands increases illness by destroying the first virus needed to combat infections and virus-causing diseases. Some argue that resistance is diminished and that repeated use of hand sanitizer exacerbates the condition.

There are times when washing your hands with soap and water is just not feasible or practical. The family may be in the car, and someone's sneezing or you are shaking hands with people and couldn't find soap and water at that time. Sometimes people don't have the mobility or equipment to wash their hands regularly, and this is the time when sanitizers can come in handy. Although they both have the same goal, they differ depending on the situation.

Many people recently saw hand sanitizers come in and becoming common because of outbreaks, such as swine flu spread in multiple countries. Hand sanitizer is an antiseptic and need not be rinsed with water. Simple to use and apply like a regular cream to your hands. It's an uncomplicated way to avoid infectious diseases like fungi, bacteria, and viruses all around. Such micro-organisms are present on polluted objects, different animals, and even certain foods. They're comfortable to hold, particularly for kids that like playing outdoors. Transmission typically takes place from source contact to a touch of the nose, eyes, or mouth. From time to time, it is best to wash your hands in between. Most people today are using foam soap than conventional solid or liquid detergent. That is because it offers a silky smooth, smooth foam. This soft feeling encourages children to wash their faces without being told frequently. Only a sufficient amount is released into the hands while dispensing foam soap, unlike the liquid variety, which tends to float effortlessly. Hand Sanitizer is a portable disinfectant that is effective at destroying the virus at any time.

Chapter 2: General Tips for Making a Sanitizer

2.1 Sanitizer's Pros, Cons and precautions

Not all Hand Sanitizer products are similar. Research published in the magazine 'Emerging Infectious Diseases' reported that not less than one brand contained 60 percent of the alcohol needed to destroy dangerous viruses and bacteria. To be efficient, the concentration of ethanol or any variance must be between 60 to 95 percent, so read the label before buying the item. Most hand sanitizer brands are the

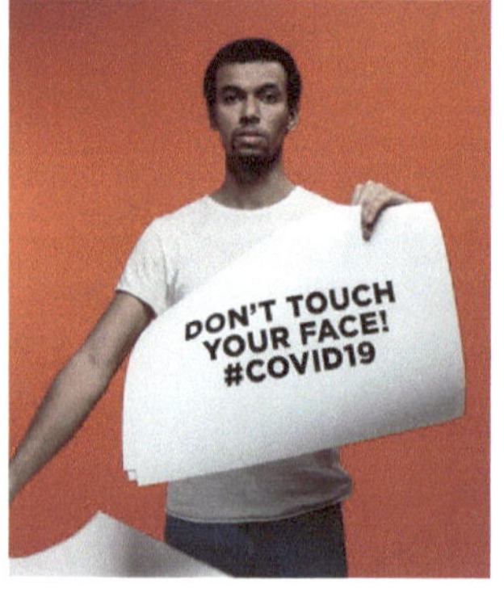

same, the same bottle, the same pump, and the same price. Instead of soap and water, hand sanitizer products are not recommended; alcohol will not penetrate dirt, so first flush dirt, blood, stool, or other specks of dust. If soap and water are not usable, friction dependent alcohol is, of course, a reasonable precaution.

When you're sneezing or immobile in your vehicle, for example, or if you miss applying contact lenses in some way, use a hand sanitizer.

Studies have shown that in telephone receivers, computer keyboards, and desktops, microorganisms are much more common, so it is advisable to use a hand sanitizer in this situation. Should not use an alcohol-based treatment until your skin shows a lot of dryness and crackling because it will only exacerbate your condition. These can lead to infection if the virus reaches the skin cracks. It is also essential to know how much to use—using enough gel to coat either side of your palms thoroughly. Generally speaking, if your hands dry out within 5 to 10 seconds, you have not been using enough. You should consider using a disinfectant in children only when appropriate, and keep gels based on alcohol out of reach of children. Please note that any substance containing alcohol is flammable and should not be stored or used close to heat or fire. When using a lighter or another lighting tool, ensure your hands are thoroughly dry.

2.2 Basic Ingredients to make a Sanitizer

It does not take much to make a hand sanitizer at home, yet a few ingredients required that can be bought locally or online. The following are the necessary ingredients that can be used to make a right, hand sanitizer, which can disinfect surfaces and destroy most germs. However, components can vary for different varieties of sanitizers from one recipe to the next.

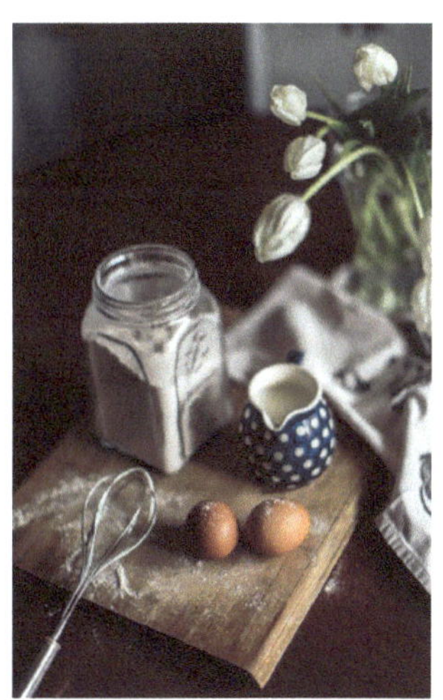

- Alcohol (isopropyl) (volume of ethanol up to 99 percent).
- Gel Aloe-Vera
- Lime.
- Essential oil.

The reasonable level of alcohol required to kill many germs is

60%, which can only be accomplished by mixing an alcohol ratio of 2:1 with Aloe Vera. This ratio would produce an efficient, microbe-killing sanitizer. This is a suggestion that comes from the Disease Control Center (CDC).

This material obeys a standard recommendation from health care practitioners on how to make a reliable and effective hand sanitizer. Isopropyl alcohol is the major component of the formula for the hand sanitizer, which can destroy a large number of germs on your hand or any surface. The formulation is a chemical compound that is colorless and combustible. Isopropyl alcohol is used in the production of several industrial and household chemicals. It is also an ingredient used in antiseptics, detergents, and disinfectants.

Isopropyl alcohol is especially useful for producing a hand sanitizer as it evaporates quickly and leaves no evidence of oil. Compared with other solvents, it is also reasonably non-toxic. The product is also ideal for cleaning electrical contacts, eyeglasses, playback/videotape ears, etc.

The Aloe Vera gel is the Aloe Vera plant's colorless, odorless jelly. It is succulent, and the leaflets contain more than 98% water in the shape of a gel rich in many valuable substances.

2.3 Making a Sanitizer with Aloe-Vera gel

If you have not been growing it in your garden, you can buy the Aloe Vera gel online, in a local store, or else make it at home. The Aloe Vera plant gel is suitable for sunburns, wounds or minor injuries, insect bites, and other skin problems. The gel also gets exceptionally moisturizing. It's simple, and it's also suggested that you grow the Aloe Vera plant at home because much of the Aloe Vera gel advertised out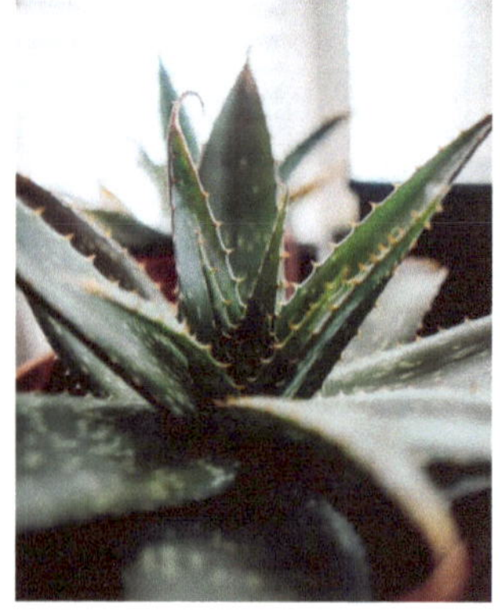 there is mixed with dyes, which is potentially dangerous You can buy the Aloe Vera leaves at a grocery store, farmer's market, or harvest it from your garden if you grow it and quickly extract the gel.

What do you need?

- A steel container that must bear-tight.
- Aloe-vera leaves
- One knife.
- A Mixer.
- Vitamin C / E pulverized (optional)

Note that the Aloe Vera gel stays about a week, so it is advised that you only process a volume you need at one time and use it all. If you plan to hold it for a longer time, you may need to add preservatives (powder form vitamin C / E). You should keep the refrigerated as well.

Direction

The development of an Aloe Vera gel takes about 20-30 minutes.

Preparation from the leaves of the Aloe-Vera

- Cut the leaves off the plant. This can also be bought from a store.
- Clean and eliminate all dirt. Stand it erect and remove the yellow-tinted resin for up to 10 minutes or more. Due to the latex found in the gum, this step is crucial.
- Clean away whatever adhesive left and scrape off the skin with a cheese grater or knife. Make your gel from the natural Aloe Vera by peeling the leave.
- You can scoop it into your mixer using a spoon. Don't enable Aloe-Vera skin particles to get into the blender.
- Mix in the gel to liquefy. Add preservatives if required. This step is only crucial if you intend to hold it for more than a week. As described earlier, vitamin C or E can be used as a preservative to prolong the Aloe Vera gel's lifetime. You can opt to add either one of those vitamins or both.
- You can add only 450 mg of vitamin C or E or perhaps for

every 65 ml or 1/4 of a cup containing Aloe Vera gel. Add the vitamin to the solution and stir again until the two items thoroughly blend.

Directions to storage

Place the Aloe-Vera gel in the refrigerator without a preservative and use it within the week. Including the vitamins significantly increases the Aloe Vera gel's shelf life for more than a week and then refrigerates it for up to two months. You will be able to keep it frozen for up to 6 months. This should be kept in an air-tight container.

Application of Aloe Vera gel

The Aloe Vera gel can be rubbed directly to repair skin issues such as sunburns, skin irritation, wounds, etc. This is an antioxidant, which can provide sunburn relief. Rich in polysaccharides, it's excellent for the skin. This is also high in the minerals and the vitamins A, C, & E. Both components have the benefit of encouraging healthy skin and speeding up recovery from problems.

Preparing the Sanitizer using Aloe-Vera gel

The essential oils that are used to make a hand sanitizer are primarily included in the formulation of its fragrance. In comparison, lemon juice can also add to the mixture as a disinfectant.

Put all the ingredients needed into a clean bowl. Most recommended is a tub with a pouring spout. Mix all with a turning stick to blend. You should then put the mixture into an air-tight bottle or an old sanitizer jar, but remember to separate the liquid from the original label. You can then label it "My home-made hand sanitizer" or ignore the labeling.

See below for its composition.

- Ethyl (two parts) of ethanol or isopropyl (85 to 99 percent ethyl).
- Gel of aloe vera (one part).
- Clove / eucalyptus / essential oil or peppermint oil

Make sure everything is prepared on a sterilized surface and in a clean spot. See to it that your hands are clean. I am using a clean mixing spoon and whisk. Use alcohol, which is undiluted. If you need to touch it wear gloves to deal with the mixture.

Chapter 3: Preparing different types of Sanitizers

The numerous hand sanitizer tips shared in this book make use of the simple formula and drive multiple variations that will suit everybody's daily routine and working lives.

To give these sanitizers more benefits for the skin, essential oils are added. Let's go ahead and try these budget-friendly, chemically-free hand sanitizers and get better grooming for yourself and your family.

3.1 Tea Tree and Lavender Sanitizer

This is a straightforward and effective recipe for creating a lavender-scented, home-made herbal sanitizer.

Ingredients:

- Ethanol or Alcohol
- Lavender essence oil
- Tea tree essential oil
- Squeeze or spray bottle
- Aloe gel

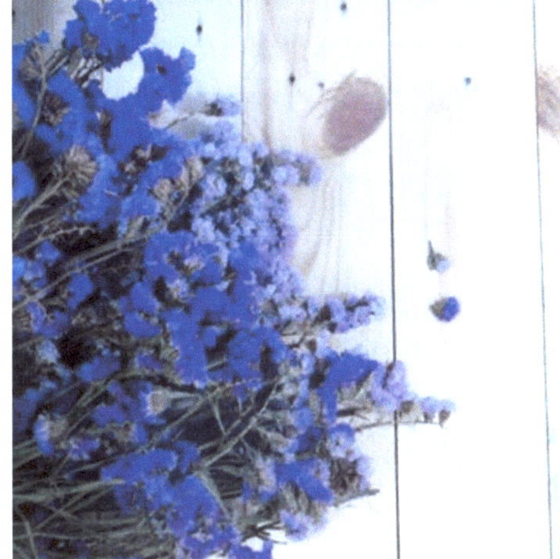

Procedure

Fill your two-third bottle with alcohol. Alcohol has to be at least 65 percent of the solution since the main ingredient is alcohol. The effectiveness drops significantly if you fall below Sixty percent.

Add around fifteen drops of essential oil from the tea tree and essential oil from the Lavender essence oil. These oils have anti-bacterial effects and combine to smell beautiful. You can also use the essential oils you like the best, too.

Fill the remaining container with aloe-vera gel. The aloe vera will make the solution more gentle on your body but don't overdo it, or you risk the blend being diluted. Just shake and put the jar into your carrier bag, ready to fight against germs.

3.2 Witch Hazel and Tea Tree Sanitizer

This method works best for those who do not want to use alcohol due to its distinctive smell and extreme body drying impact. The witch hazel is a convincing alcohol substitute and is extracted from the Witch Hazel shrub's steam distilling of the leaf and wood.

Components:

- One cup raw aloe vera gel (preferably without additives)
- Half tablespoon witch hazel
- Mixing bowl
- Spoon Funnel
- Plastic bottle
- Thirty drops tea tree oil.
- Five drops essential oil, like lavender.

Procedure:

Take a pan and pour Aloe Vera gel, tea tree oil, and witch hazel and blend all combined. If the mixture is too small, add another aloe vera spoon to emulsify it. If you think that's too dense to your liking, add another witch hazel spoon.

Stir the lavender oil into it. Because the tea tree oil odor is already substantial, go easy on the essential oils that are added. Four drops is a must, but pour it in 1 drop at a time if you want to add more.

Funnel the combination into the dispenser. Place the funnel inside the jar and pour the sanitizer into it. Fill it, then place it on the cover until you can use it. If you're producing so much of a hand sanitizer and you can't fit it all in the bottle, save the remaining sanitizer in a tightly sealed cover container.

3.3 Citrus Hand Sanitizer

This organic hand sanitizer is impressive because it is produced with all-natural ingredients, and because of the mixture of plant oils it is obviously antiviral and anti-bacterial; which ensures you get strong bug-killing and sanitizing effects as a typical hand sanitizer product, but you don't probably spread poisonous chemicals on your hands.

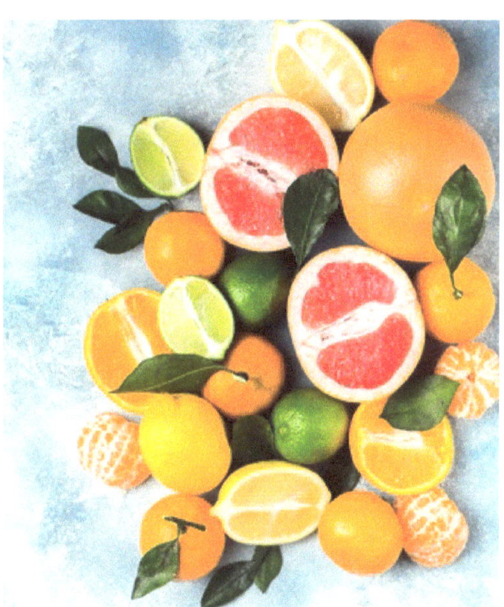

Ingredients:
- Five drops of essential lemon oil
- Five drops of vitamin E oil
- Two tablespoons witch hazel(with aloe vera or vodka)
- An ounce of spraying flask
- Five drops of essential orange oil
- Five drops of essential tea tree oil

Procedure:
Mix vitamin E oil with hazel or vodka and other oils in a plastic container. Place the sprinkler tightly on as well and spin well to blend for 15-20 seconds.

After done, open the bottle and add water up to the tip. Remove the sprayer, then shake for 15-20 seconds again. Tribute!

You can also print the sticker and add it to the bottle. Print the label on a standard paper if you don't have sticker sheets lying around, and then use transparent packaging tape to stick the sticker to the bottle utilizing the tape.

Spray your hands-free if you like; they must have a touch of a deep scrub. Clean your hands until dry.

3.4 Peppermint Oil Sanitizer

It is also a natural but alcoholic hand sanitizer.

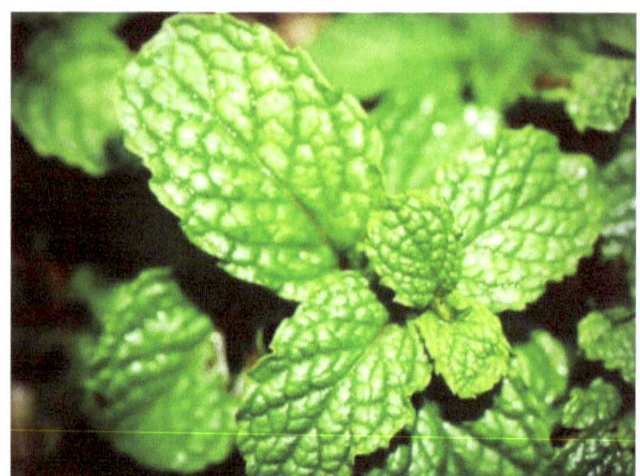

Ingredients:

- Half tablespoon aloe vera gel
- Five drops of tea tree oil
- 15 drops of fresh peppermint oil
- One teaspoon alcohol rubbing
- Two cups distilled water

Instructions:

Put the essential oil, tree oil, and alcohol in a glass cup, and mix it. Include the aloe vera gel and blend well. Then add the water and blend again until done. Put the hand sanitizer through a funnel into tiny, clean squirt bottles. Place away from direct sunlight in a cool spot. You need to shake before using it.

3.5 Cinnamon Oil Sanitizer

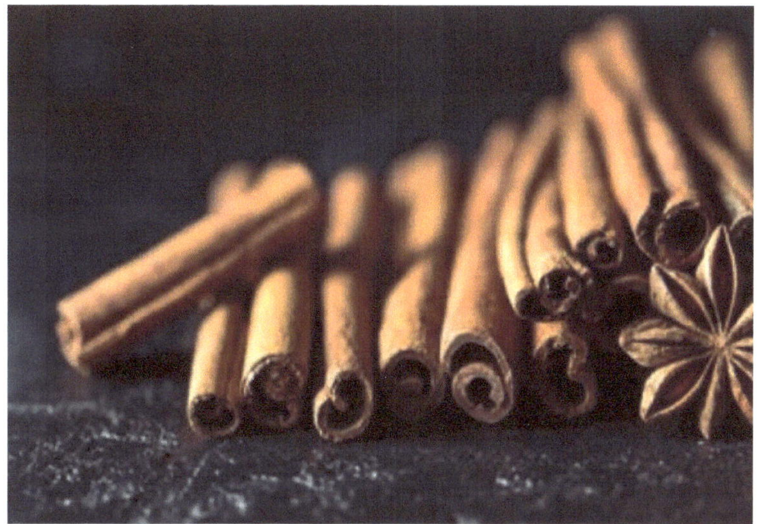

Cinnamon is a spice of the genus Cinnamomum, derived from the inner bark of many tree species. Cinnamon is rich in a medicinal agent with essential properties. It is filled with antioxidants and protects against inflammation.

Ingredients:

- Five drops of vital cinnamon oil
- Half tablespoon aloe vera gel
- Two cups filtered water
- Five drops of tea tree oil
- One tablespoon alcohol rubbing

Instructions:

Put the essential oil, tree oil and rubbing alcohol in a glass cup, and mix to blend. After that, add the water, aloe vera gel, and blend well until combined. Put the hand sanitizer via a funnel into a sterile bottle. Place away from direct sunlight in a cool spot. Always shake before using it.

3.6 Caraway Sanitizer

Caraway is a spectacular spice that has long been used in herbal medicine and cooking. This tiny, brown pod, while sometimes mistaken for seed, is indeed the dried fruit of the caraway plant.

Components:
- Five drops of liquid caraway oil
- Two cups filtered water
- Five drops of tea tree oil
- One teaspoon alcohol rubbing
- Half teaspoon Aloe-vera gel

Instructions:

Put the alcohol, essential oil and tree oil in a glass cup, and mix to blend. Insert the aloe vera gel and add the water. Mix them until ready. Put the hand sanitizer through a funnel into a bottle. You can use it, but remember to shake every time before use.

3.7 Hydrogen, Glycerol and Tea Tree Sanitizer

Here is another fast and simple recipe for making an effective hand sanitizer. The beautiful thing about this recipe is that it would be less sticky on your hands because there is no aloe vera. I have explained it to make a large scale sanitizer, which you can also sell to others.

Ingredients
- 3% hydrogen peroxide, which is used to inhibit the growth of contaminating enteric bacteria in the mixture and is not the main ingredient for hand antiseptics.
- Plastic blending paddles
- Weighing tubes and quantifying jugs
- Plastic or metal funnel
- 420 ml Glycerol (98%), which serves as a body lotion.
- 155 ml Sterile distilled water
- An alcoholmeter
- Two gallons of ethanol or 2 gallons of isopropyl alcohol (> 95%).

Procedure:

This is a commercial formula that can be packed in 10-liter transparent plastic cans with screw-threaded clamps to prevent spillage. Let's just see how to plan it progressively.

Spill the alcohol into the container or big bowl up to the graded mark. Using the measurement cylinder, insert Hydrogen peroxide. Using a measurement bottle, add the glycerol. Since glycerol is very viscous and sticky, some pure distilled or cold boiled water should be rinsed and then dumped into the container/tank. Now spill in 15 drops of essential oil from the tea tree. The bottle/tank is then filled with pure distilled water up to the 10-liter level.

Put the lid or the top cap on the tank/bottle as soon as possible when you finish; this will avoid any evaporation. Blend the solution with a soft shaking. Wait 75 hours before use.

3.8 Douglas Fir Sanitizer

Douglas fir is known as the most common evergreen tree in Southern British Columbia and the Pacific Northwest. Several people use Douglas Fir extract for skin since, when applied topically, it provides cleaning, antibiotic, and purifying effects.

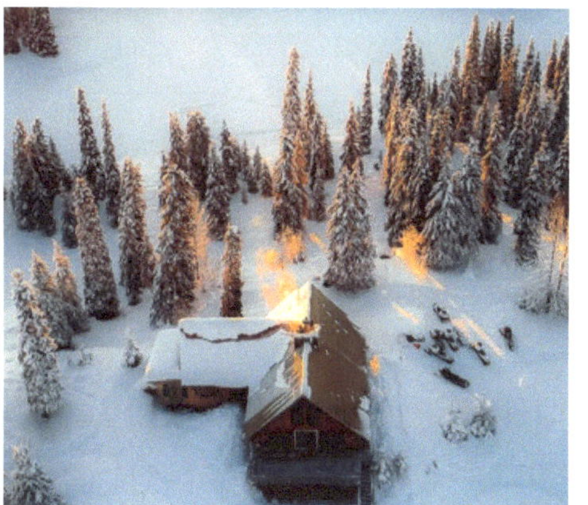

Contents:

- Half table teaspoon aloe vera gel
- 15 drops of essential Douglas fir oil
- Five drops of tea tree oil
- One tablespoon alcohol rubbing
- Two cups filtered water

Instructions:

Put the essential oil, tree oil and alcohol in a glass bowl, and mix to blend. Include aloe vera gel, add water, and incorporate it until ready.

Put the hand sanitizer via a funnel into tiny, clean squirt bottles. Store off direct sunlight in a cool spot. Care to shake before any use.

3.9 Eucalyptus Oil Sanitizer

Eucalyptus is a perennial herb, commonly used for its medicinal qualities. It is an anti-inflammatory agent by nature. Eucalyptus oil is a natural repellent for insects primarily due to its amount of eucalyptols.

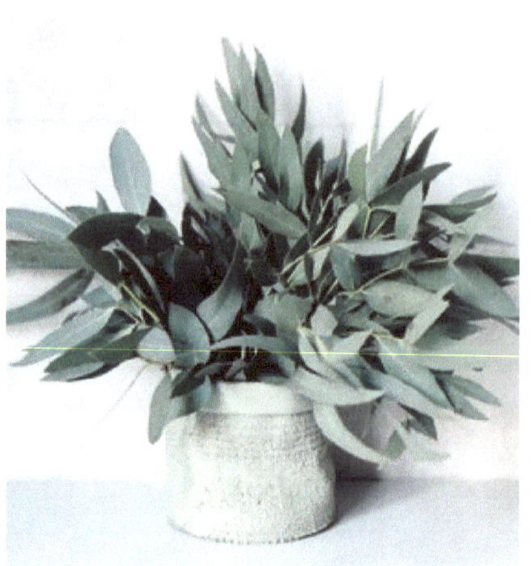

Materials:

- Fifteen drops of essential eucalyptus oil
- 2 cups distilled water
- Five drops of tea tree oil
- One tablespoon alcohol
- Half tablespoon aloe vera gel

Instructions:

Put the essential oil, tree oil and alcohol in a glass cup, and mix to blend. Add the aloe vera gel, water, and blend until mixed. Put the hand sanitizer via a funnel into slim, clean squirt bottles. Carry away where ever you need it.

3.10 Get Maximum benefit from a Sanitizer

Last year hand disinfectants became more common because of H1N1 shocks. Though they are inexpensive, they cannot provide as much protection as you think if they are not used properly. The efficacy of this drug in reducing illness depends on the ingredients and the method of use. Here are three things to use and how to use a hand disinfectant. Ethyl alcohol is a well-known giant killer in hand disinfectants, but not only that, and any alcohol gel is doing what we need. East Tennessee State University performed several tests and found that testers left 50 percent of the virus in the hands of a product containing 40 percent alcohol. To get rid of most germs, they agreed they needed medication with at least 60 percent alcohol, according to the Association for Infection Control and Epidemiology Professionals.

If you wear rings on your fingers, use detergent to wash them. The rings are the perfect

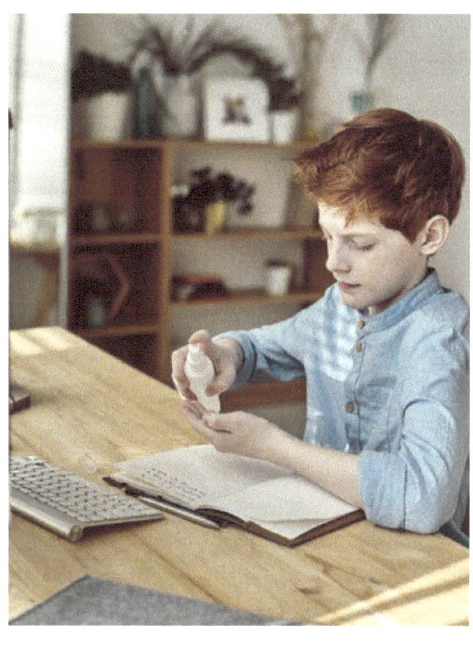

hiding place for viruses and pathogens, so put the virus on fresh hands, if you wash them before using hand disinfectant. Hand disinfectants do not harm precious metals like gold but do use soap and water to disinfect your hands if you have jewelry.

Hand sanitizer with the right amount of alcohol is very powerful, but to remove all the germs, you need to make sure you cover all your side. Only missing a tiny spot will leave a thousand viruses. You need to start with a quarter-size disinfectant and work it in a curve between your fingertips, palms and the back of your hand, and finish by making sure you touch all the fingers. The Federal Drug Administration (FDA) and the Center for Disease Control (CDC) suggest washing your hands with good quality soap and warm water for at least 21 seconds, scrubbing on your wrists and under your thumb. Many of us don't thoroughly wash our hands to prevent the virus from spreading. If it's not possible to wash hands with soap and water, they suggest using a hand disinfectant, known as a hand cleaner with an alcohol content of at least 60 percent, to be effective against the transmission of viruses. Make sure to carefully read the bottle, as many alcoholic hand sanitizers have a lower alcohol content to avoid drying and damage to the skin. To prevent harmful transmission, alcohol is necessary, but it's raw on the surface. Some have added Aloe and vitamin E to cope with alcohol's detoxifying effect, which helps strengthen and soothe the skin. Another part which is not very well known is the dimension.

Dimethicone used in cosmetics of high quality is an emollient used to treat dry and rough skin and to avoid it. The key to dimethicone is that not only does it help heal, but it also prevents irritation of the skin. It can be used in rash ointment rash, as well. The hand disinfectant comes in the form of a spray, paste, and gel. The drying of the gel takes a little longer than the foam, and the alcohol is not entirely effective until it remains on the skin for 15 seconds, so I prefer the gel to the foam for this reason.

There are many other chemicals used in antiseptics for antivirus characteristics, Triclosan, which has been filed by the Environmental Protection Agency (EPA) as a pesticide, and Benzalkonium Chloride, which experiments have shown support for antibiotic resistance. For several years alcohol has been used safely, and I choose to follow the accepted guidelines of the FDA and the CDC.

We come across viruses everywhere. There is both good and bad virus, and yes, both of us need it. A good virus is known as 'resistant flora' is a helpful virus found in the skin and intestines. A healthy virus helps to prevent the lousy virus from rising and from getting sick. Lethal viruses or 'pathogens' cause diseases, viruses, and parasites.

While, as advised by the FDA and CDC, the hand disinfectant kills both useful and harmful viruses, I'd rather know those potentially lethal viruses won't attack me. The CDC recommends good hand sanitizer or antiseptic hands before cooking, eating, taking care of the infant, supporting the elderly or compromised health, prescribing medications, and wearing contact lenses. Having used the toilet, changing diapers, collecting garbage, collecting pet garbage, coughing, sneezing, and handling raw foods, we suggest you wash or use an antiseptic side.

The cold and flu season is inevitable, so do your study and get prepared, but note that proper hygiene sanitizer and hand-cleaning, as suggested by the FDA and CDC, should be practiced in our everyday lives to avoid many harmful viruses and potentially fatal diseases.

CONCLUSION

Carrying a moisturizing hand sanitizer is a good idea, specifically during the flu season. People usually acquire the horrific flu virus by contacting infected people or surfaces. It's especially troubling about this is that you can't even tell if the doorknob of the supermarket you've just entered, the deck on the train, or the item you've just passed in the food store, are infected before the symptoms appear up.

The easiest way of avoiding the flu outbreak is always to be aware and stay safe by using sanitizers.

REFERENCES

- Ashworth, B., n.d. *How To DIY Your Own Hand Sanitizer*. [online] Wired. Available at: <https://www.wired.com/story/how-to-make-hand-sanitizer/>.
- Healthline. n.d. *How To Make Your Own Hand Sanitizer*. [online] Available at: <https://www.healthline.com/health/how-to-make-hand-sanitizer>.
- Popular Science. n.d. *How To Make Your Own Hand Sanitizer And Help Fight COVID-19*. [online] Available at: <https://www.popsci.com/story/diy/diy-hand-sanitizer/>.

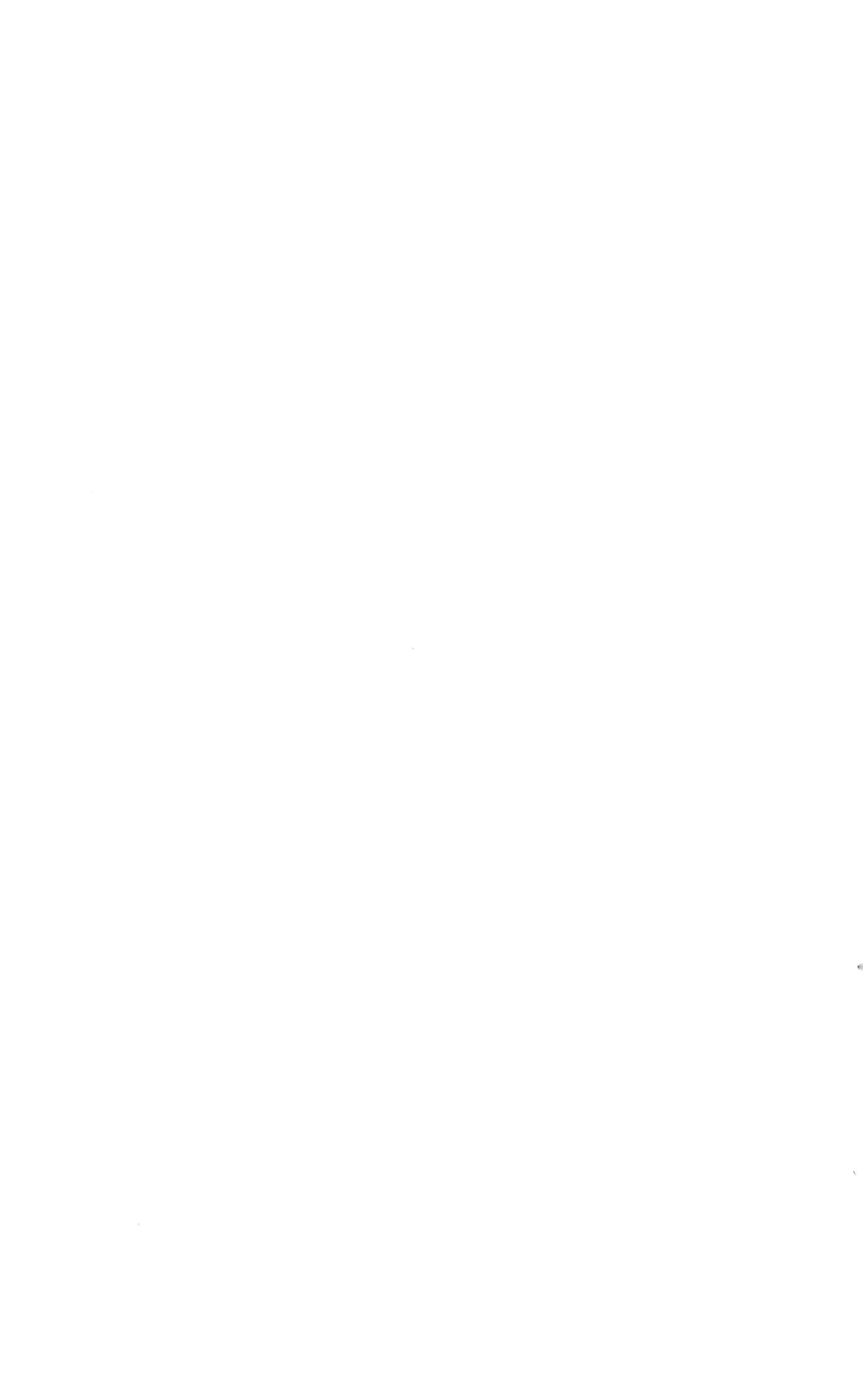